"Balan
Achieving a Youthful Hormone Balance

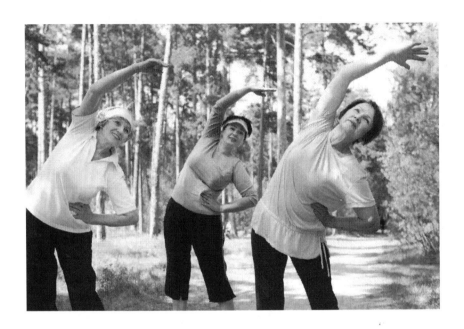

By
Dr. Tammy Post

"Start your amazing, wonderful, fabulous life of having your hormones balanced, feeling good, sexy and back in CONTROL!"

Dedication

To all those who have struggled with "not feeling right", knowing that your hormones are out of balance... and have fought the good battles but feel like you are losing the war, I dedicate this book to you. It's not your fault and you are not alone.

I am grateful to God for what I call, "allowing things to happen for me and not to me", as these personal experiences and trials with my own hormone imbalance issues have led me to be able to help you.

To all those patients who have taught me, through precious trial and process, what to do and what not to do, I thank you that others can learn from your journey.

For information about permissions to reproduce selections from this book or to purchase copies for educational, business or sales promotional use, contact:

Better Living Rx
4201 SW Lilac
Bentonville, AR 72712
800-479-6435

All rights reserved. No part of this book may be used or reproduced without written permission except for personal use. This book is intended for healthy adults age 18 and older. This book expresses the author's personal medical opinion and is not medical advice or to be substituted for medical advice. Please consult with your own physician regarding new exercise, nutrition or supplementation program or questions about your health. As individuals differ, individual results will vary. The statements in this book have not been evaluated by the Food and Drug Administration. The author and any of her affiliated LLCs do not accept any responsibility for any injury sustained as a result of following the advice or suggestions contained within the content of this book.

"Balancing Act"
Achieving a Youthful Hormone Balance

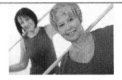 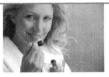 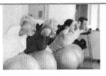

<u>TABLE OF</u>

CONTENTS

Introduction

How do you know it's your hormones? It's <u>not</u> just about hot flashes. How do you know your hormones are out of balance?

If you are reading this book you have probably, at one point in time or another, asked if your hormones could be out of balance. Maybe a spouse, friend or family member has asked you cautiously but sincerely, *"Have you thought about getting your hormones checked, honey?"*

Maybe you have had weight gain that has not been typical or mood changes that you just can't explain...

Maybe you even went to your doctor and asked to have your hormones checked. Maybe they did a little blood work or maybe they didn't, but told you, *"You're fine."* Or, *"It's not your hormones"*. Or worse, *"You're just depressed"* Or, *"You just need to reduce stress, eat less and exercise more."* Maddening, right?

So many patients are frustrated because intuitively they know it's a hormone problem. And guess what, if you're asking that question or suspect it, IT IS!!!!! Hormones drive every process in your body and if you don't feel right or out of balance, I guarantee you, IT IS

YOUR HORMONES OUT OF BALANCE. But it's not your fault and you are not alone. So let's get you started on the path to figuring out how to regain your life and balance.

To start uncovering where and how severe the imbalance may be, I have my patients fill out a quite lengthy questionnaire which helps me to understand them better. It gives the best insights as to how to use the labs in combination with symptoms to decide a course of action for balancing their hormones.

It also helps you assess the severity of your hormone imbalance and address the list of symptoms or issues that may help you monitor and keep track of your hormone balance.

Take a look at the information sheet on the next page. As you can see, I have patients check the box if they are having symptoms and then circle the level they are experiencing: Mild, Moderate, or Severe.

If you're having severe symptoms now, print out this page, answer the questions and email your responses to info@betterlivingrx.com.

You can get started even before you finish reading this eBook.

- ☐ (Mild, Mod, Severe)   PMS (premenstrual syndrome) issues, such as cramps, nausea, breast tenderness, headaches, and/or irritability 1-2 weeks before my period
- ☐ (Mild, Mod, Severe)   Difficulty falling asleep or staying asleep
- ☐ (Mild, Mod, Severe)   Fatigue or loss of energy especially in the afternoon
- ☐ (Mild, Mod, Severe)   Frequent bouts of irritability and depression
- ☐ (Mild, Mod, Severe)   Frequent anxious feelings, anxiety attacks, or heart palpitations
- ☐ (Mild, Mod, Severe)   Achy or stiff joints, especially in the morning
- ☐ (Mild, Mod, Severe)   Gaining weight, especially around the middle
- ☐ (Mild, Mod, Severe)   Losing weight is more difficult than in the past
- ☐ (Mild, Mod, Severe)   Pain with intercourse
- ☐ (Mild, Mod, Severe)   Inability to have orgasm, decreased sensitivity, or sex drive
- ☐ (Mild, Mod, Severe)   Vaginal dryness
- ☐ (Mild, Mod, Severe)   Crave sweets, carbohydrates or alcohol.
- ☐ (Mild, Mod, Severe)   Hair or skin that is dry, fragile, or thinning

- ☐ (Mild, Mod, Severe)   Losing height, diagnosed w/osteoporosis, broken or fractured bones
- ☐ (Mild, Mod, Severe)   Recurrent yeast or urinary tract infections.
- ☐ (Mild, Mod, Severe)   Irregular menstrual periods.
- ☐ (Mild, Mod, Severe)   Hot flashes or night sweats.
- ☐ (Mild, Mod, Severe)   Missing the outer third of your eyebrows
- ☐ (Mild, Mod, Severe)   Frequent headaches or migraines
- ☐ (Mild, Mod, Severe)   Fluid retention (rings fit tight or shoe size increased)
- ☐ (Mild, Mod, Severe)   History of cysts on ovaries
- ☐ (Mild, Mod, Severe)   Male distribution hair growth (facial hair, male pattern balding)
- ☐ (Mild, Mod, Severe)   Problems with acne or rosacea
- ☐ (Mild, Mod, Severe)   Heart racing or irregular heartbeats felt
- ☐ (Mild, Mod, Severe)   Hot or cold intolerance
- ☐ (Mild, Mod, Severe)   Constipation or diarrhea
- ☐ (Mild, Mod, Severe)   Frequent bouts of abdominal bloating or gas
- ☐ (Mild, Mod, Severe)   Skin rash or new onset allergies

Chapter 1 - The Journey

So why me? Why am I the one to help you on your journey?

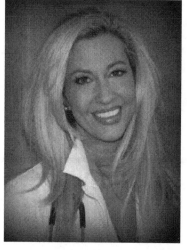

I was born in a small town to a family with a lot of chronic illness issues. I was skinny as a child and never really had much trouble managing my weight. Right from the beginning of my female adult experience, I experienced terrible menstrual cycles, heavy and irregular. Pain doubled me over and I spent many nights in the bathroom crying and rocking from the pain. Birth control pills were prescribed and only made me feel worse. Years went on. I was diagnosed with ovarian cysts, tumors, PCOS (polycystic ovarian syndrome) and endometriosis. I bled more days than not. I had many abnormal pap smears and procedures.

I struggled with infertility for thirteen years. During this time I did get pregnant but had a miscarriage at three months, which was devastating! No one had any answers or could tell me what was happening. I felt very alone and scared. Afraid to ever try to get pregnant again. The

• Copyright © 2016 Dr. Tammy Post/ Better Living Rx

menstrual issues just seemed to get worse. I don't know how I made it through medical school and residency with all the issues I had with pain and bleeding.

Finally, after thirteen years, I got pregnant unexpectedly. This time I carried the baby full term. Although, I had severe complications and almost died in the ICU. I had gained over seventy pounds with my pregnancy from the steroids they had me on just to survive and was miserable. I was still wearing my maternity clothes for months after the baby was born. Breast feeding helped drop some of the weight, but I was always hungry.

The periods resumed and were heavier than ever. I had a right side pain that sent me to the doctor for an ultrasound. The ultrasound showed I had several fibroid tumors and a mass on the right ovary. The gynecologist suspected cancer and so I did the only thing I knew to do. Have a hysterectomy.

After my hysterectomy, I didn't suffer from periods, but new problems cropped up, the hot flashes began. I started having adrenal/stress issues and my thyroid started to fail. I was gaining more weight. Almost eighty pounds!

I am a doctor and I really had no clue how my own body really worked or how to fix it. Sure, I took biology and physiology, but no one ever told me what I really needed to know about hormones and the impact they have on the human body.

One day a patient came to my clinic, dressed professionally and quite eloquent with her words. *"Do you prescribe bioidentical hormones?"* she asked matter-of-factly.

"Bio what?" I asked.

"You know," she paused *"natural hormone therapy... like Suzanne Somers uses".*

I had no idea what she was talking about, so I looked at her more intently, leaned in, and said, *"Tell me more."*

She proceeded to tell me about natural hormone therapy and all the benefits of it. I was astounded. My jaw dropped as she talked about a world out there that was completely foreign to me. I thought hormone replacement therapy was bad, very bad. I thought it was only to be used for the woman who was soaking in sweat constantly or homicidal/suicidal.

I had received so much faulty information in medical school from pharmaceutical companies. They continue to feed us faulty information.

Until that point, I believed a woman didn't need progesterone if she didn't have a uterus. I was taught there was only one way to take hormone replacement therapy and only a couple of different options or doses.

I told my patient I knew nothing about what she was talking about, and I promised her I would find out. I try to keep an open mind about alternative therapies although many physicians don't because there is already so much to learn and know. Why add more? These physicians ask, "If there is no evidence-based research behind it (or at least that's what big pharmaceutical companies would have us believe), isn't it better to prescribe a pill?" Some doctors cattle forty or more patients through their halls a day. That doesn't leave much time to look into alternative therapies. *I feel very differently about this and for this reason I vowed to look into "bioidentical hormone therapy".*

I googled Suzanne and soon had unlocked a door to a world I never knew existed. That was eight years ago. So, what was the outcome?

• Copyright © 2016 Dr. Tammy Post/ Better Living Rx

I started on bioidentical hormone therapy (and I prescribed it for that patient, too). I lost over sixty pounds and escaped night sweats and hot flashes! My mood was stable for once and I was sleeping again. I put testosterone in the prescription and actually got a libido back that might have saved my marriage. I felt better than I had felt since those nasty periods started when I was a teenager.

I learned that my hysterectomy was probably not necessary. The abnormal pap, fibroids, and endometriosis found at the time of my surgery were all a product of my massive hormone imbalances. I learned my heavy periods were from the excess estrogen I was storing, when I unknowingly put on an extra 10 lbs in college. From this and more, I have learned patients do not have to suffer and have unnecessary procedures, surgeries and rely on big pharmaceutical companies' answers to these issues.

So my journey began. I thank that woman every day for intriguing me with something new. I didn't know it that day, but I had embarked on a journey. Looking back, this time was the beginning of my understanding of everything you are reading here.

Over the past twelve years I have treated thousands of patients, I have seen patients lose hundreds of pounds, but more importantly people have transformed before my very eyes. Marriages have been healed from the ravages of hormonally imbalanced women AND men. I have been given a gift to be able to help people through this journey.

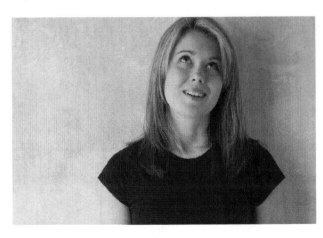

I have sought out every aspect of metabolic realignment I could and this is the simplest presentation I have come up with. The principles are really quite simple, although the nuances can be tricky. You will need a physician on your side willing to go the distance and pay attention to the details.

Why YOU? Consider this...

When there is a sudden change in cabin pressure during an airline flight and the oxygen mask drops down, what are you supposed to do? You put the mask on yourself, FIRST! *Why? Because if you don't take care of yourself first, you can't take care of or help anyone else.* If you lose consciousness you can't put the mask on your child or dependent loved one.

You have to put yourself first or you can't help anyone.

This may go against everything you think or believe, but if you are not healthy you lose your effectiveness with your children, your spouse, your work and even yourself.

Understanding hormones is about taking care of yourself so that you can take control and make a difference in the lives of everyone around you. When you make positive changes in your life, your children will learn from your healthy choices.

Start today by choosing to be healthy and take control of your life.

Copyright © 2016 Dr. Tammy Post/ Better Living Rx

Chapter 2 - How Did I Get Like This?

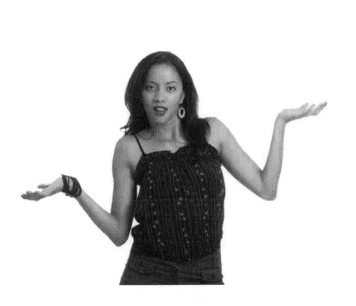

Well, let's start by saying that it is not your fault. You may have made some decisions that lead to these issues but probably made those decisions unaware of what you were doing to your body.

This is an appropriate answer for the question that many patients ask: "How did I get like this?" Day after day the average American participates in an all-out onslaught on their own health. Overwork, physical and mental overstrain, sleep deprivation, noise pollution, late hours, surgery, medications, injuries, inflammation, pain, toxicity, ingestion of chemicals, poor diet filled with packaged and processed non-nutritive foods, electromagnetic fields, poor digestion, blood sugar issues,

Copyright © 2016 Dr. Tammy Post/ Better Living Rx

environmental xenohormones, allergies, and the list goes on and on. We did not even talk about emotional stressors. Oh, we just did.

All of these insults to our systems lead to endocrine disruption and hormone imbalances. When we chronically don't take proper care of our systems, they begin to malfunction. Your body may require more of one hormone in a certain instance. When that hormone increases over a period of time, others will begin to decrease leading to imbalance. Allow this strain of the system to go on long enough and you have a full scale war going on inside of you, and you are the benefactor of all the suffering.

Female hormone imbalance is rampant in our country.

It affects nearly all women at one time or another in their lives. Indirectly, it affects us all! It is reported that 60% of American women suffer from PMS. It is apparent that major interference with female hormone balance is occurring on a daily basis. A major cause of these changes is estrogen dominance. Estrogen dominance occurs when the estrogen level increases, or when the progesterone levels decreases. Balance between these two hormones is essential for proper function of the female hormone system and the body.

Research has shown that many women will have months where they do not ovulate. When the woman does not ovulate, the corpus luteum does not form, therefore no progesterone is produced. If such a situation occurs again, a progesterone deficiency will develop resulting in estrogen dominant state and all of the issues that ensue with estrogen dominance. One reason for a women not ovulating is the chronic stress response and adrenal fatigue. When adrenal function becomes compromised, hormone imbalances result. Several problems can develop, one of which is abnormal cycles, hormone patterns, long or short periods, and no ovulation.

Estrogen most often takes the blame for various symptoms related to female hormone imbalances.

Ask stated earlier, proper testing is the only way to truly determine the status of the female hormones and the imbalances themselves.

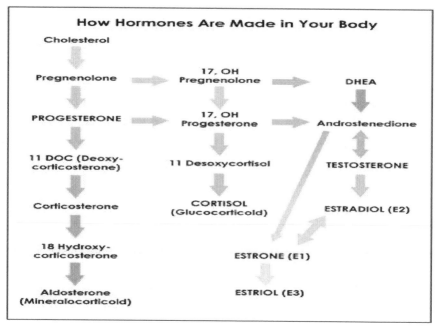

*Notice E1, E2 and E3 and the arrow directions

The above diagram shows the importance of having a healthy amount of cholesterol in the body. Cholesterol is the precursor molecule to the sex steroid hormones. Enzymes convert these hormones from precursor molecules to other forms. Constantly your hormones are in transition.

Why Are We All So Scared of Estrogen?

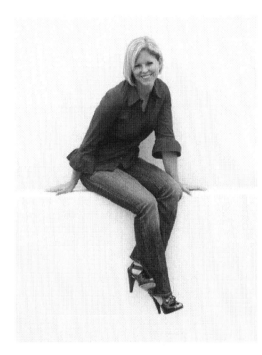

- Until 2002, mainstream physicians routinely prescribed conventional SYNTHETIC hormone replacement therapy (HRT) in order to alleviate menopausal symptoms such as hot flashes, mood swings, decreased sexual desire, vaginal dryness, and difficulty sleeping, as well as to prevent heart disease and osteoporosis.

- In 2002, however, the results of a landmark study, the Women's Health Initiative (WHI), identified dangers associated with conventional hormone replacement therapy in women. More than 160,000

Copyright © 2016 Dr. Tammy Post/ Better Living Rx

women participated in this observational study. Conventional HRT side effects included a 26% increased risk of breast cancer, 29% increased risk of heart attack, 41% increase in risk for strokes, and a doubling in risk for blood clots relative to the untreated group. Moreover, women receiving conjugated equine (horse-derived) estrogen experienced a six-fold increased risk for uterine cancer.

- Reasons for this include synthetic hormone, route of delivery and unopposed balance from faulty thinking (i.e. no uterus, no progesterone needed).

- Beginning in perimenopause and continuing throughout menopause, the production of progesterone tends to decline more rapidly than that of estrogen. If the progesterone to estrogen ratio is unbalanced, favoring excess estrogen, a woman may become susceptible to an increased risk of fibrocystic breast disease and other health problems.

- Factors contributing to estrogen dominance include: Exposure to estrogen-mimicking chemicals found in herbicides, pesticides, petrochemicals (e.g., BPA, bisphenol A) and PCB's (polychlorinated biphenyl's) used in some cosmetics, glue, plastic, and other modern materials.

- Copyright © 2016 Dr. Tammy Post/ Better Living Rx

- Concern about cancer is an important reason why more aging women do not restore their hormones to youthful levels. Hormones like estrogen and testosterone affect cell growth and proliferation. Does that mean aging women should simply accept hormone deficiency as a part of "normal" aging?

If estrogen caused breast cancer, then we would expect to see very high rates in young women of childbearing age, with a dramatic decline after menopause. This has not been observed. In fact when you are 25 years old your risk of breast cancer is 1 in almost 20,000. By the time you are 85-years-old your risk goes up to 1 in 9!

In a healthy young woman, progesterone serves as a counterweight to estrogen during the menstrual cycle. Estrogen levels rise during the first half of the cycle and progesterone levels rise in the middle.

Progesterone's job is two-fold: 1) to prepare the uterus for implantation with a healthy fertilized egg, and 2) to support the early stage of pregnancy. If no implantation occurs, progesterone levels drop until another cycle begins. Studies have shown that progesterone has anti-proliferative effects on breast cancer and leukemia cells. Breast cancer is 5.4 times more common in pre-menopausal women with low progesterone levels than with favorable levels (Cowan 1981). Data suggest that while bioidentical (i.e., natural) progesterone does not increase risk of breast cancer, synthetic progestins used in conventional HRT do.

Natural progesterone has also demonstrated neuroprotective properties. One study called for more attention to progesterone as a "potent neurotrophic agent that may play an important role in reducing or preventing motor, cognitive, and sensory impairments (in both men and women)" .

The difference in chemical structure is obvious...

Progesterone (Natural, human)

Medroxyprogesterone acetate (Synthetic)

The difference in structure can promote a pregnancy (pro-gestation) and keep a woman who has had difficulty carrying a pregnancy to term, versus synthetic which will cause a miscarriage (DEATH) to a fetus!

• Copyright © 2016 Dr. Tammy Post/ Better Living Rx

Chapter 3 - Hormones 101

So What Are Hormones?

Remember in college, the basics start with the "101" Classes. So here, we go, let's start with the basics and unravel the mystery of hormones and demystify them as well as debunk the myths like **ESTROGEN IS BAD and ALL HORMONES ARE ESTROGEN.**

The word hormone comes from the Greek word *hormān* meaning to "urge on" or "impulse."

Hormones are more than just estrogen. When most people think about hormones they think of estrogen and immediately fear comes to mind. Pharmaceutical companies have manipulated estrogen and made it unsafe, convinced doctors they have the only option, and created mistrust of "hormones".

Amazingly, on a daily basis patients tell me their doctor put them on estrogen after having a hysterectomy and told them they didn't need progesterone because they didn't have a uterus anymore. Let me explain why this is amazing to me.

• Copyright © 2016 Dr. Tammy Post/ Better Living Rx

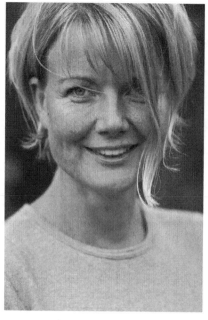

Progesterone has so many more uses than just preventing lining buildup in the uterus. It's like saying that you don't need shoes because you're not wearing any socks, but as we all know shoes have more functions than just covering up your socks. When patients tell me they are scared of hormones, I take a lot of time to undo the damage that big pharmaceutical companies have done. Their unnatural manipulation of the basic hormone structure given to women in unhealthy doses and distribution forms is not good.

We all have hormones.

Some of my emphysema patients tell me they don't want to go on oxygen because they are afraid they will get addicted to it. HELLO?! We are ALL addicted to oxygen! We cannot live without it! Some people need a little purer form or an increased concentration of it to help the heart and lungs work more efficiently.

Pharmaceutical companies know hormones cannot be patented. God invented them. He has the ultimate patent. By the way, you can't patent oxygen either. For marketing purposes and sales, they figured out if they changed the structure, they could patent the new compound, and sell it for a lot of money. Problem is the new compound is just different enough to cause problems. The amount is "one size fits all" and the route through the gastrointestinal tract and liver filtering creates inflammatory proteins causing all sorts of problems from joint aches to blood clots and, worse yet, cancer.

Remember, all hormones work in concert to balance each other. One is not more important than another. One may be more abundant at certain parts of the circadian rhythms, but they are always in balance.

Did you know you are a walking, talking, shopping bunch of hormones? Hormones control everything we are and do!

Estrogen – Makes us "girly"; induces puberty in females and facilitates the menstrual cycle in preparation for fertilization. Less known functions include libido, breast health and enhances female traits and characteristics.

Progesterone - Helps maintain menstrual cycle. It is more than just a hormone of uterine balance, however,

Copyright © 2016 Dr. Tammy Post/ Better Living Rx

because it helps with mood balance, sleep, and appetite or weight gain just to name a few of its purposes.

FSH - Causes menstrual cycle to START. This is a great marker as a blood test if you question whether or not you are in menopause. As the ovaries start to decompensate FSH increases in the feedback loop. If your periods are irregular this will help clarify menopause.

LH - Triggers ovulation and creates corpus luteum. In guys, it triggers production of testosterone.

Insulin - Comes from the pancreas and regulates sugar or carbohydrates in the blood stream. It does this by removing sugar from the blood stream, lowering the blood sugar level and stores the glucose in various cells (usually fat). Therefore, when this hormone is elevated for long periods of time it stops working effectively and you are likely to gain weight.

Glucagon - Is produced in the pancreas and functions to raise very low blood sugar. Glucagon is also used in diagnostic testing of the stomach and other digestive organs.

Testosterone - Makes guys look like "guys." It enhances and builds muscle (anabolic). It also maintains bone density, regulates hair growth, and maintains healthy libido or sexual interest. In males, it is primarily secreted from the testes, and YES females have testosterone too! It comes from the ovaries and sometimes from the adrenal glands. Males make about ten times as much as females, although females are more sensitive to its effects.

Thyroxin - Usually abbreviated as T4. Thyroxin is a pro-hormone meaning that it is inactive and must be converted to triiodothyronine (T3) or the active, more potent, form. It does this conversion in the target tissues and works to regulate just about every physiological process in the body including but not limited to growth, development, metabolism, body temperature and heart rate. It also helps as a lipid modifying agent affecting weight gain and loss.

TSH – Is released from the pituitary gland in the brain and stimulates production of thyroid hormones. It is a very sensitive blood indicator for thyroid function.

Aldosterone – Comes from the adrenal gland and regulates sodium and potassium in the kidney. It increases blood pressure by retaining sodium. It may have further indications for hearing loss and ringing in the ears.

Anti-diuretic Hormone - Regulates water retention and blood pressure.

Ghrelin - produced mainly by the lining in the stomach and cells in the pancreas and stimulates hunger. It is considered the counterpart of the hormone leptin. Highly regulated by adequate sleep.

Leptin - (Greek *leptos* meaning thin)- which is made in fat cells and induces satiation when present at higher levels. Leptin plays a key role in regulating energy intake and energy expenditure, including appetite and metabolism.

Melatonin - "hormone of darkness" released from the pineal gland in the brain when the level of light is decreased and helps induce sleep. Closely balanced with leptin and ghrelin.

And these are just a few!

Chapter 4 - Understanding Yin and Yang of Hormones

The body is constantly trying to stay in balance. The hormones are intimately connected and in constant communication with each other. They are what Chinese philosophy calls "Yin and Yang". I believe that the universe itself is bound by balance and counterbalance. Yin and Yang encompass the all-in-one belief that the earth and the universe, even, are all one system. There is no superiority. Only balance.

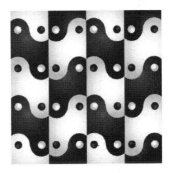

Each yields to the other without question. It takes a human mind to mess up the balance. Harmony is the balance of the system and any deviation can drastically disturb it.

We live in a society where more is better. When we accept balance, we know this cannot be true. In every decision, there are pros and cons. This is the balance that the universe maintains over us. When we accept this concept the body becomes an orchestra with a conductor. It is then we can understand how balance becomes the key issue.

• Copyright © 2016 Dr. Tammy Post/ Better Living Rx

The concept of the universe and the moon ties us to something even bigger than ourselves. Think about it... lunar cycles. There is no coincidence that the moon takes approximately 28 days to orbit the earth and this about the time of a "normal" menstrual cycle. In fact, the same root word in Latin is menses (to measure and menstrual) meaning month and echoes the moon's importance to measurements of time.

Also, of interesting note, every 223 months (also called a Saros cycle) the sun, moon, and moon's nodes align in the same relative angles to each other. This happens about every nine years. Then every 56 years the elliptical position of the north node of the moon moves and the sun's relative position will shift resulting in alternating solar/lunar eclipses.

Is it coincidental that every nine years humans experience monumental changes? A nine-year-old child starts the hormonal changes that trigger puberty. An eighteen-year-old human starts the cycle of starting to establish societal roles. Thirty-six-year-old humans in our society are at the peak of child rearing and at forty-five, many humans are experiencing their "mid-life crisis". Then in our fifties, we start the cycle of menopause (yes, men do too) and then in our sixties, we start to experience significant increases in age-related diseases and become eligible for Medicare.

So, if we deny the Yin-Yang theory and fail to realize the balance of the universe, we make many mistakes in our metabolic balance. Technologic advances have led us to many ways we can counterbalance these lunar cycles. Pharmaceuticals now make chemicals that interfere with our hormonal balances and many unsuspecting people who ingest them on a daily basis. *(More on xenoestrogens and petrochemicals later.)*

Let me now describe a few patterns within the human body that clearly show the Yin-Yang balance. What comes to mind? Okay, probably estrogen. Well, if the Yin is estrogen than the Yang would be progesterone.

Progesterone's role in balancing estrogen is well established and the feedback loop with one another is classic hormone science. What about insulin? If insulin is Yin, then its Yang would be glucagon which has opposite effects but maintains the same goal of glucose metabolism and storage in body. While insulin lowers blood sugar, glucagon works to raise it.

Thyroid hormone balance (both active and inactive forms) is achieved through feedback with TSH (thyroid stimulating hormone) from the brain. Leptin and ghrelin are Yin-Yang hormones of hunger and satiety (fullness) and closely regulated by sleep.

Some hormones even have two names, like growth hormone balance. The Yang to growth hormone is the hormone somatostatin and it is also called GHIH or growth hormone-inhibiting hormone. It also has the name somatotropin release-inhibiting factor. That name alone establishes its Yin-Yang nature. Its unique properties are in its ability to regulate growth and to regulate (feedback for inhibiting and releasing) many other hormones to stay in balance.

Some hormones are balanced by the substrate or materials available within a closed system. Example: Calcium concentration feeds back with a hormone called parathyroid hormone to keep calcium concentration balanced in the blood stream, but parathyroid hormone also has a Yang called calcitonin, a hormone that lowers calcium levels in the blood.

The biggest balancing act in the human body is the balance between the blood stream content and storage or usage of materials in the tissues. This balance is orchestrated starting with the HPA or hypothalamus/pituitary/adrenal axis. Like a fine tuned orchestra, every instrument has its

• Copyright © 2016 Dr. Tammy Post/ Better Living Rx

own place and sound. When one is out of balance, all of the music sounds bad.

The HPA (hypothalamus-pituitary-adrenal) axis is no different and drives everything you do. Every thought. Every action. Hormones are all driven very intricately by a feedback loop intertwined with one another and delicately balancing the whole body. The conductor, in this case, is "stress" and is responsible for deciding the players and the hormone's roles with each other.

Cell Communication

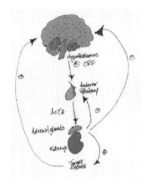

Cell communication is an important key and hormones do that. There are two major classes of hormones: PPA (protein, peptides, amino acids) and steroid hormones. PPAs bind to receptors on cells and alter their behavior by sometimes opening channels into the cell and sometimes closing them or going straight to the nucleus (powerhouse of the cell) to turn genes off and on. Steroid hormones go into cells and exert their power there, while PPAs work from the surface to trigger a cascade of events.

Did you know you actually need your cholesterol? All steroid hormones come from the cholesterol molecule.

Since steroid hormones are made from cholesterol (or fat molecules), it can easily slip into cell membranes that are fat soluble. To keep them from just plopping into any cell they usually catch a ride on "carrier proteins", like "hormone taxis".

Steroid hormones are further grouped into five categories depending on what receptors they bind to. These are: glucocorticoids (sugar), mineralocorticoids (electrolyte balance), androgens (think testosterone), estrogens, and progestogens. Vitamin D is a close cousin to a steroid hormone.

These are important basics because it explains why the feedback loops are so important and balance is essential, but enough with science terms.

Chapter 5 - What are "Bioidentical Hormones?

When women have been out of balance for a while, 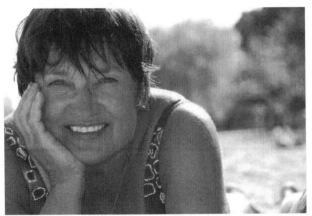 often times it is necessary to use some degree of hormone therapy to get them back in balance. This has been the basis of what I have done and they way I have helped women achieve balance.

As I learned on my journey about natural bioidentical hormones and knew how they helped me, I wanted to share that with my patients as well. I did my homework, learned from the gurus and began implementing therapy. I have continued to learn and tweak the process over the years.

They don't teach this stuff in medical school or residency so I had to learn it from anywhere I could and through working with patients over the years have come to deeply appreciate the value of bioidentical hormones and how they can help when you have severe imbalance or deficiency.

So, what are bioidentical hormones exactly? They are the hormones that are identical to the human body's hormones. I often use the term 'designer' or "individualized" is brought in for discussion, we are talking about the fact that one size does not fit all. The doses are tailored to our individual needs. People need different clothes sizes; our human hormones can vary quite a bit. Even environments affect our hormones through different levels of stress.

Bioidentical hormones are manufactured in the lab to have the same molecular structure as the hormones made by your own body. By contrast, synthetic hormones are intentionally different. Drug companies can't patent a bioidentical structure, so they invent synthetic hormones that are patentable.

It's so unbelievable to me that bioidentical hormones have been around for years, although most doctors have never heard of them. Big pharmaceutical companies that have expensive patented synthetic hormones would like to make sure they never do. The biggest problem is that one size does not fit all when it comes to hormone therapy and most of the traditional synthetic hormone therapies are only that. One or two, maybe three different doses.

By contrast, the bioidentical or designer hormones are dosed specifically to a patient's blood or saliva hormone levels but mostly by symptoms or concerns. It's important to have your doctor order lab tests (saliva or blood) to

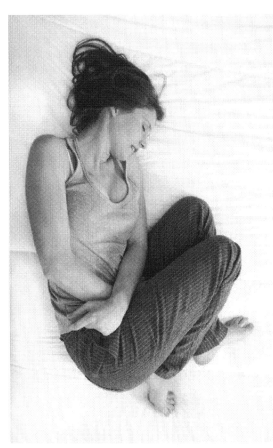

establish baselines, rule out serious disease/tumors, and to assess success of absorption into the system from time to time. Not every person needs hormone therapy. When they do though, many medical studies suggest that bioidentical hormones are safer than synthetic versions. It is often possible to rebalance hormones without the use of hormonal supplementation by using nutritional supplements, gentle endocrine support, and dietary and lifestyle changes.

Even with this foundation, a minority of women will need to add prescription-strength hormone supplements to get complete relief, at least through a transition period. We recommend they use bioidentical hormones, preferably in a compounded form personalized to their needs by an experienced practitioner.

There is no substance we introduce into our bodies that is not without potential side effects. Even water can be dangerous when you drink too much. There has been a lot of press around the negative statements from the WHI (women's health initiative) studies on the effectiveness and health risks of HRT, but it is important to remember that these studies were based on synthetic/equine-based hormones taken by mouth.

The WHI was launched in 1991 and consisted of a set of clinical trials and an observational study, which together involved 161,808 generally healthy postmenopausal women. The clinical trials were designed to test the effects of postmenopausal hormone therapy, diet modification, and calcium and vitamin D supplements on heart disease, fractures, and breast and colorectal cancer.

The hormone trial had two studies: the estrogen-plus-progestin study of women with a uterus and the estrogen-alone study of women without a uterus. In both studies, women were randomly assigned to either the hormone medication being studied or to placebo.

I, personally, feel the benefits of bioidentical natural hormone therapy are more than just symptom relief.

I rarely run into a woman who is not symptomatic from some sort of hormonal imbalance symptoms. Regardless, I feel the benefits of preventing osteoporosis and keeping the mind, skin and blood vessels youthful is of upmost importance. With all the controversy around hormones and breast cancer, the question comes up, *"What about bioidentical hormones if a person has had breast cancer?"* The pendulum has swung so far that very few doctors will prescribe any type of HRT, synthetic or bioidentical , for women who have had breast cancer or even a family history of breast cancer.

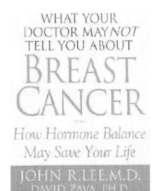

I recommend you read Dr. John Lee's book, *"What Your Doctor May Not Tell You About Breast Cancer".* He also has several other great books that I consider to be my "bibles" of hormone education study.

Chapter 6 - Hormone Myth-Buster: Not All Estrogens Are Bad

Estrogen often gets a "bad rap" because we have come to relate estrogen with cancer thanks to a landmark

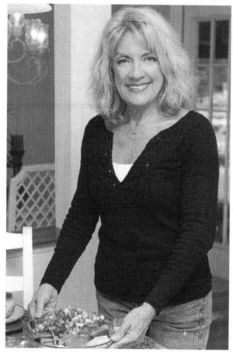

study done in 2002 that has created fear, frustration and confusion in the world of hormone therapy. The biggest issue in this study was that they used "synthetic" hormones (not the same as natural hormones and gave them in not only an ineffective route but potentially dangerous and did not explore the need for balance of all of the hormones. Three fatal flaws of hormone balance protocols that I embrace, teach and prescribe.

Let's explore these issues further.

Premenopausal women produce three biologically active estrogens, estrone (E1), estradiol (E2), and estriol (E3). Estradiol is the most abundant estrogen produced and both estrone and estradiol are potent estrogens. Estriol is considered a weak estrogen. Although little scientific data supports the claim, it has been postulated that estrone is a "bad" estrogen and may be the cause of estrogen's cancer-causing properties, while estriol is a "good" estrogen and may protect against cancer. Estradiol is probably neutral.

Oral estrogens, not estrogens given by systemic routes (patch, skin cream, vaginal cream, under the tongue), are converted into estrone with potential negative effects for the patient. Oral estrogens, because they are metabolized by the liver, likely exert different effects than systemic estrogens which are not metabolized by the liver.

So, yes, women who have had breast cancer might consider this alternative if they are symptomatic with menopause or pre-menopause. It is thought estrone is a "bad" estrogen and may be the cause of estrogen's cancer-causing properties. Estradiol is probably neutral, but helps significantly with hot flashes.

Over 13 million women were on some form of synthetic HRT before the initial studies were published. When the studies came out millions quit "cold turkey". I can only imagine all those women and their symptoms returning. Many stayed on synthetic HRT, but live in fear of the consequences and hormone replacement therapy side effects.

Many of those women were unnecessarily placed on antidepressants as pharmaceutical companies and doctors gained alliance to position those drugs as substitute products for lack of hormone balance. Most of 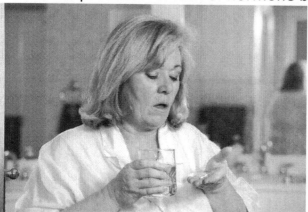 these women were not depressed and now have been exposed to a new set of potential side effects.

The majority of studies published to date have used synthetic HRT, specifically Premarin and Prempro. Both of these forms are usually take in pill form or orally. Studies have shown levels of CRP (c-reactive protein) are increased with intake of oral estrogen. CRP is a pro-inflammatory blood protein associated with increased risk of heart attack and stroke.

Very few have involved or reported anything about bioidentical hormone replacement therapy. Oral estrogens are converted into estrone with potential negative effects; not estrogens given by transdermal or through the skin routes (patch, skin cream, vaginal cream, under the tongue).

Oral hormones, with a focus on estrogen, are metabolized by the liver. This is known as first pass metabolism. When this happens a normal process occurs that creates "inflammatory proteins". These proteins can cause many different types of inflammation in the body. Of most concern are the blood vessels with a risk of a heart attack or a stroke.

When a route through the skin is chosen, this first pass metabolism by
the liver is bypassed and goes straight to the tissues that need it.
This is why we choose creams and gels.

Although I do not recommend oral estrogen, there were problems with the WHI study that no one really talks about. For one thing, the women in the WHI studies were on HRT after menopause while the most common therapeutic use of HRT is for perimenopausal symptoms. Also, the higher risks are small in absolute terms, the increases in relative risk are significant. To take heart attack as one example, the WHI data taken as a whole indicated that out of 10,000 women on Prempro, an extra six would have a heart attack each year compared to women not on Prempro. That may not seem like a substantial risk, but it is a much greater relative risk. The WHI study indicated that the overall increase for women on Prempro for breast cancer was 26%, for heart attack

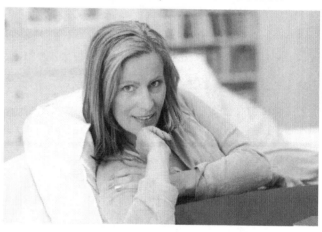

29%, for stroke 41%, for blood clots 100%, and for Alzheimer's or dementia over 100%.

Many of the top problems in women's health are on that list. And, even if there is not as great a risk of heart attack as originally supposed, for women closer to menopause, the overall risk-benefit ratio is significant.

Thankfully, there are good alternatives to synthetic HRT.

Dr. John Lee, author of *"What Your Doctor May Not Tell You About Menopause"*, a pioneer of bioidentical hormone therapy stated that there are three rules to hormone replacement therapy. The first rule is to use hormones only if you "need" them (based on lab values or symptoms). The second rule is to use bioidentical hormones and never synthetic, and the third rule is to only use hormone replacement in dosages that create hormone balance. Many women don't even require hormone therapy. Sometimes symptoms can be controlled by a program of core nutritional and endocrine support.

Many women who switch over from oral synthetic estrogen to natural forms of estrogen and progesterone undergo a transition period. It is as if the body's hormone receptors have been primed by the synthetic molecules and have trouble recognizing other forms, even a woman's own. Sometimes, the transition can take four to six weeks. I often start slowly reducing the synthetic dose (not quitting cold turkey from the oral form) as I start with a low dose of bioidentical estrogen and titrate up slowly as the synthetic is getting out of the system. If you stop too abruptly, you may experience extreme hot flashes or other symptoms may flare due to the change in the hormone receptor status.

There are a number of nutritional supplements available that can be extremely helpful in this process. A medical-grade multivitamin combined with calcium, magnesium and essential fatty acid (fish oil) is critical in diminishing the number and severity of symptoms that occur while one is stopping HRT and afterward. Regular exercise can make a huge difference in terms of the number and intensity of postmenopausal or perimenopausal symptoms.

The use of black cohosh as well as soy (80–100 mg of isoflavones a day) may also help abate the symptoms of hot flashes. Be sure to avoid genetically modified soy; choose products labeled "Non-GMO." Soy has also been shown to be helpful in reducing the risk of heart disease; some studies have demonstrated improved bone density; and most recently, studies have shown its ability to decrease the response of insulin in the body, which is particularly important for those who are insulin resistant or diabetic.

Of concern for me is the fact that Wyeth, the manufacturer of Premarin and Prempro, petitioned the FDA in 2005 to restrict the availability of compounded

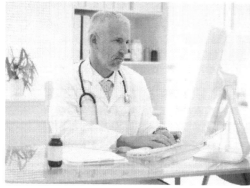

"bioidentical " hormones.

There are a few things you should know about bioidentical hormones. One of them is that they are usually compounded. This means that they are formulated based on the precise specifications of a doctor who prescribes them rather than in predetermined doses.

There are many medications that are compounded; bioidentical hormones are just one of the many. Some people say that there is an issue with compounded prescriptions and that they are not FDA approved. The FDA doesn't approve any compounded products, for any condition, because those products can't be standardized. And, therein lays the beauty in the art of compounding.

One size does not fill all when it comes to hormone therapy. I prescribe the lowest and most exact dose formula on symptoms to control those symptoms most effectively.

Compounding can also be useful for patients who are allergic to an additive FDA-approved product. Because compounded products don't go through the FDA approval process, they don't bear the same warnings as other hormone therapy.

Just because the process is not approved does not mean the actual ingredients are not approved. They absolutely are. It is important that since compounding is a precise science that patients look for accredited compounding pharmacies listed on the web site of the Pharmaceutical Compounding Accreditation Board

(PCAB). Since these accredited pharmacies can be hard to find, due to the stringent rules, patients should ask compounding pharmacies what types of quality assurance procedures are in place. Also you will need to ask for information on side effects and warnings because these may not be included when prescriptions are compounded.

It is not completely necessary you use compounded hormones. There are FDA-approved "bioidentical " drugs available.

The biggest reason for using compounding is the customization of doses. Another reason to use compounding would be if someone has allergies to ingredients, or intolerances to doses, in commercially available products.

There is no reason to think bioidentical compounded products would have a different safety profile than the FDA-approved ones. You must be careful as some compounding pharmacies have gotten warning letters from the FDA for false and misleading claims about safety and other benefits.

Compounding pharmacies can formulate products into many forms including tablets, capsules, creams, gels, lozenges, suppositories and more. Compounding pharmacies create products from one or more active ingredients. The United States Pharmacopeia (USP) is the recognized national formulary and offers guidance for compounding. Ingredients, according to the USP, must meet quality standards; such as: pharmaceutical grade, reagent grade or even food grade. The active ingredients and inactive ingredients are specified by a licensed health care physician with a prescription.

The healthcare practitioner specifies ingredients and doses intended to meet the individual needs of their patients. For example these pharmacies can combine multiple bioidentical hormones of various strengths into one compounded medication. The prescriber will also specify the type of formulation to use. Flavoring can be added to formulations to make them more palatable, if desired.

The greatest success comes from an individualized approach. When warranted, we prescribe a precise dosage of bioidentical estrogen, testosterone or DHEA that is made up at a compounding pharmacy to alleviate individual symptoms and target specific issues to the individual. Each patient is then monitored carefully through regular follow-up. Treatment and adjustments should be based on symptoms and quality of life issues more than blood hormone levels. Lab tests (saliva or blood) are best to use to establish baselines, rule out serious disease/tumors, and to assess success of absorption into the system.

"How long will I need to be on Hormone therapy?"

The answer to this depends on how long you have symptoms or the body has issues consistent with hormone deficiencies. For some this is a few months, for others many years. I believe when your body is in balance your adrenal glands can make all the same hormones that your ovaries can, so adrenal health is very important if a patient wants to get off any type of supplemental hormone therapy.

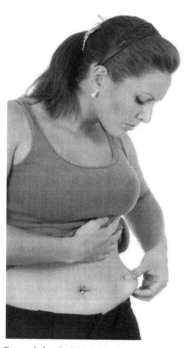

I have also come to learn about "leaky gut and nutrition", that all hormone imbalance starts in the gut so if you address and repair those issues while giving attention to any other hormone imbalance like adrenal or thyroid issues then you won't need

• Copyright © 2016 Dr. Tammy Post/ Better Living Rx

hormone supplementation.

Your body can make and regulate hormones perfectly if the conditions are right. EVEN after a total hysterectomy!

I also get asked about having periods after menopause. It is not necessary for a postmenopausal woman to have periods if using bioidentical hormones properly. When postmenopausal women use small doses of bioidentical hormones, they rarely, if ever, have periods. Nor do they have the risky endometrial buildup in the uterus which is what makes it important to have periods.

Estrogen stimulates the buildup of uterine tissue, but there's no need to take that much estrogen to feel healthy and balanced. Since fat cells create estrogen, women who are heavy may not even need to use supplemental estrogen.

Dr. Lee's recommendation was always to use the lowest dose possible of any hormone supplementation. Usually this was 15 to 30 mg of progesterone daily, and the lowest dose of estrogen that would either clear up estrogen deficiency symptoms or show normal levels on a saliva hormone level test. This improves health and well-being, but doesn't put a postmenopausal woman back into the same hormonal milieu I had when I was menstruating every month.

When you take progesterone in a pill form, most of it goes directly to the liver, where up to 80 percent of it may be dumped, but not before creating a variety of byproducts (metabolites). Thus, it's necessary to take 100 mg of progesterone in pill form to get 20 mg into your cells.

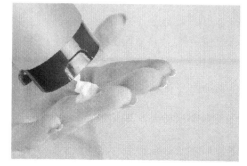

If your liver happens to be working less efficiently on a given day, and excretes less of the progesterone, it's easy to experience overdose side effects, such as sleepiness and bloating.

These side effects often have women running for more estrogen to wake themselves up again.

What they really need to do is use progesterone cream, which is a much more efficient delivery method. If you put 20 mg on your skin, virtually all of that will be in your bloodstream within a matter of minutes.

Chapter 7 -
How Should I Get Tested?

I usually start with a full panel of hormones that not only include the ovarian hormones: estrogens (estrone, estradiol, estriol), progesterone, testosterone but also adrenal, thyroid and more specific testing as indicated by symptoms. I always relate the tests to the symptoms in a "functional" analysis which is part of the art of this science of helping achieve hormone balance.

Saliva testing has become one of the most popular ways to assess the hormone levels in your tissues. Although some insurance carriers do not pay for it; these tests can be more affordable than blood tests in many cases. If you have ever done one, you know that collecting saliva can be quite a challenge, especially a tube full!

Saliva testing is a convenient, inexpensive, and above all, accurate means of testing steroid hormones.

Scientific studies have shown a strong correlation between steroid hormone levels in saliva and the amount of hormone in the blood that is active or "bio-available." Saliva is an ideal diagnostic medium to measure the bio-available levels of steroid hormones active in the tissue. It is this fraction of total hormone that is free to enter the target tissues in the brain, uterus, skin, and breasts.

Copyright © 2016 Dr. Tammy Post/ Better Living Rx

Saliva testing can be done anywhere, anytime, unlike testing that relies on blood drawn in the doctor's office, which makes it harder to obtain samples at specific times (such as in the early morning) or multiple times during the day. In addition, hormones in saliva are exceptionally stable and can be stored at room temperature for up to a week without affecting the accuracy of the result. This offers maximum flexibility in sample collection and shipment. Several of the steroid hormones can be tested in the saliva including, estradiol, estrone, estriol, progesterone, testosterone, DHEA-S, and cortisol.

Each person is different and the whole person and hormonal chemical make-up and balance are unique. The doctor must take into account all the different complexities of an individual's hormone make-up and balance and work with what the person has in their environment to maximize the hormonal balance.

Chapter 8 -
Path to Balance

The hormonal health of any woman depends upon the delicate dance of progesterone and estrogen. Estrogen is meant to be the predominant hormone in the first half of the menstrual cycle and progesterone the predominant one in the second half. However, for most women in the industrialized world this is not the case.

There are many causes of hormone imbalance, but at the base of the problem is something called Estrogen Dominance - which means there is too much estrogen and not enough progesterone present in the body. There are many symptoms that result from having low progesterone levels.

What follows is a look at some of the common ways in which medicine and industry have tampered with the natural balance of our hormones. Women have used these products blindly at the cost of our hormonal balance, overall health, and longevity. Some of these may be obvious to you, while some may come as a surprise. Either way the hormonal imbalances that result should not be taken lightly. They contribute to the rise in cancers, especially breast and ovarian cancers, heart disease, depression, PMS and more.

The common causes of hormonal imbalance and estrogen dominance:

- Artificial hormone replacement therapy (The Pill and traditional HRT)
- Environmental poisons
- Non organic and estrogen pumped animal products
- Stress
- Cosmetics (chemicals in them that mimic estrogen in the body)

Progestins and progestogens (artificial progesterone) found in synthetic HRT (hormone replacement therapy), infertility medications and birth control pills are highly toxic
to the body, resulting in some of these known side effects:

- miscarriages
- migraines
- heart disease
- high blood pressure
- cancer
- depression
- and, of course ... lowering the true biologic levels of progesterone.

- Copyright © 2016 Dr. Tammy Post/ Better Living Rx

Here are some the ways that industry has tampered with the same delicate hormonal balance.

Chemicals such as pesticides mimic the hormone estrogen. Fifty-one chemicals have now been identified as hormone disruptors. Approximately 2 billion tons of pesticides are used annually the world over. In undeveloped countries, the use of pesticides is still largely unchecked and ... guess what? *That is where we get a lot of our food supplies.*

It's plain to see why this is wreaking havoc on our bodies. It is this fact that has led many people to switch to an organic diet. Other chemicals that cause the same challenges are DDT, dioxin and PCB's (polychlorinated biphenyls.) Dioxin is the by-product of the manufacture of chemicals using chlorine and includes:

- disinfectants
- dry cleaning fluids
- pesticides
- drugs
- plastics – polystyrene and cling wrap in particular

PCB's are used in:
- lubricants

Copyright © 2016 Dr. Tammy Post/ Better Living Rx

- plastics
- paints
- varnish
- inks

Commonly called petrochemicals, they contain high levels of xeno-estrogens. Xeno-estrogens basically mean they mimic estrogen in your body. They fill up all the estrogen receptor sites in your body; even the good estrogen can't get through to perform its role properly. This results in hormone imbalance. This is why many people have moved over to household cleaning products that don't contain these chemicals and are environment friendly.

Non-organic animals that are slaughtered for our food chain are fed estrogenic steroids to fatten them up. These estrogens go straight into our blood stream causing a further rise in estrogen levels and more importantly they are further putting your hormones out of balance.

As if all of the above were not enough, stress also plays a big part in reducing our levels of progesterone which results in ... too much estrogen.

Here's how: Progesterone is the "mother of all hormones." It is the precursor and essential raw material out of which the body created ALL THE OTHER

HORMONES. As the precursor to all the other hormones in the body, the adrenal glands and adrenal hormones are no exception. If you encounter a mildly stressful situation your body draws on its progesterone to produce the hormones (adrenal corticosteroids) to counteract it.

These are the hormones that protect against stress. BUT, if your body is in a constant or permanent state of stress it can't provide enough progesterone to be converted into anti-stress hormones and the result is adrenal exhaustion and no left over progesterone for other normal body functions.

You can change your life! You can restore balance.

You can combat aging and ill health effects starting today. You must find someone knowledgeable about hormones and who will listen to you and your situation 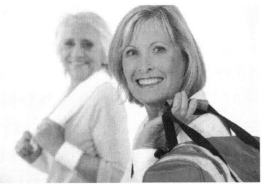 and find the right solution that fits only you. Bioidentical hormones are already in our bodies. Patients who need oxygen supplementation often tell me that they are afraid they will get "addicted" to oxygen if they start using a machine.

This is so silly because we are all addicted to oxygen. We need it every second of every day. The same holds true with our hormones. We need them every second of every day and using natural hormones to supplement deficiencies cannot possibly cause you to become addicted to hormones. I am always careful to use the term supplementation, not replacement.

You do not simply stop making sex steroid hormones after your ovaries fail and shrivel up. You still make hormones from your adrenal glands, the little guys on top of the kidneys, although, in much smaller amounts than if you have healthy active ovaries. Supplementing your body to bring you back in balance makes sense in many circumstances.

Chapter 9 -
Hormones, Disease and aging *(husbands this is about you too!)*

Aging and disease are just the consequence or process of your hormones getting out of balance. It's funny we say, "Oh, I'm just getting older... what do you expect?" But what we really should be saying is, "What the crap happened to my hormone balance?!?!!?"

With this decline, in both, men and women we are looking at feeling bad, wrinkling up to heart disease, stroke, osteoporosis and chronic inflammatory and neurodegenerative disorders among the many consequences.

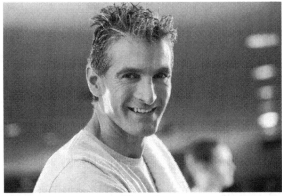

What about the guys? Men have problems with decreasing testosterone, as well. Mainstream medicine's ignorance regarding how to effectively and safely treat testosterone decline is not only annoying but downright detrimental in my opinion. Most people are in a state of denial about declining hormone levels. A 30 to 40-year-old man is often shocked when his blood test results uncover strikingly low testosterone levels. I see it in my practice all the time, especially, if they are overweight, smoke, are diabetic or have a history of marijuana use or take cholesterol medication.

Testosterone is required for optimal transport of excess cholesterol from our tissues and blood vessels to our liver for processing and disposal. In the testosterone-deficient state, reverse cholesterol transport is compromised, and excess cholesterol cannot be removed from the arterial wall.

One of the biggest barriers for testosterone supplementation is the fear of prostate cancer. However, this need not be a fear because hundreds of clinical trials have shown that low testosterone is more of a risk factor than high testosterone levels and men with low testosterone levels have an increased percentage of prostate cancer-positive biopsies. It has been shown that as free testosterone levels decline in aging men, their PSA levels sharply increase. Even though it is clear that testosterone does not cause prostate cancer, I still educate my patients on the how balance is key with estradiol and progesterone levels as well as addressing overall hormone issues and inflammation states.

Another problem with hormonal imbalance is that excess abdominal fat is a major culprit in many men

• Copyright © 2016 Dr. Tammy Post/ Better Living Rx

and women with high estradiol levels. Excess body fat, particularly in the abdominal region is a major factor in imbalanced estrogen metabolism. Abdominal obesity increases aromatase activity, which increases estradiol, which in excess causes more abdominal fat. A negative feedback loop is established and health suffers as a result. Reducing abdominal fat will reduce the excessive estradiol levels as well as natural aromatase inhibitors like zinc, DIM and occasionally I will use pharmaceutical aromatase inhibitors if the estradiol levels are greater than 30 in men.

Estradiol levels correlate significantly to body fat mass and more specifically to subcutaneous abdominal fat. Subcutaneous abdominal fat acts as protection to keep toxins from our internal organs but also as a secretory gland, often producing and emitting excessive levels of estradiol into the blood. One's waist circumference is a highly accurate prognostic measurement of future disease risk. Excess estradiol secretion is at least one of the deadly mechanisms associated with the difficult-to-resolve problem of having too much abdominal fat.

Symptoms of excess estrogen include:

- having too much abdominal weight
- feeling tired

- suffering loss of muscle mass
- having emotional disturbances

Many of these symptoms correspond to testosterone deficiency as well.

Both men and women need estrogen to maintain bone density, cognitive function, and even to maintain the inner lining of the arterial wall (the endothelium). Both men and women with declining hormone levels are at increased risk of osteoporosis, a condition that means your bones are weak, and you're more likely to break a bone. Since there are no symptoms, you might not know your bones are getting weaker until you break a bone. A broken bone can cause disability, pain, or loss of independence.

With the decline of the female hormone estrogen at menopause, usually around age 50, bone breakdown markedly increases. For several years, women lose bone density two to four times faster than they did before menopause. The rate usually slows down again, but some women may continue to lose bone rapidly. By age 65, some women have lost half their skeletal mass.

Hormones are essential to life function. Without hormones, we cannot survive. They control most aspects of all of our bodily processes. Without hormones, a woman cannot get pregnant. Without hormones, a man cannot get a woman pregnant. Without hormones, a child cannot grow. Without hormones, we cannot sleep. Without hormones, we cannot properly fight infection or the effects of stress. The list goes on.

Think of our body system's functioning like a system of checks and balances. Various hormones control the cascade of functions that occur. Most hormones have an agonist/antagonist type of relationship with another

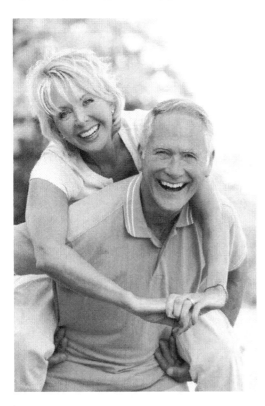

hormone. For instance, estrogen and progesterone are both steroid hormones that are dependent on each other. Cortisol and DHEA are adrenal hormones that have such a relationship.

Balance is the key to proper hormone function and therefore, bodily function. When hormones become imbalanced, trouble follows. The "system of checks and balances" of our endocrine system will normally respond in an opposite direction. If one hormone improperly rises, another hormone will usually fall. Imbalance is the result.

By the time a woman enters menopause, she may have already experienced two decades of hormonal imbalance. During the postmenopausal period, when sex hormone levels decrease significantly, aging women are at increased risk of the following diseases: heart disease, osteoporosis, Alzheimer's, dementia, among others.

Heart disease. Heart disease is the leading killer of American women. The risk for postmenopausal women is equal to that seen in men. Menopause can cause elevations in blood pressure, low-density lipoprotein (LDL) cholesterol, total cholesterol, triglycerides, as well as homocysteine levels, C-reactive protein, and interleukin-6 (an inflammatory cytokine), which are all associated with estrogen deficiency. At the same time, high-density lipoprotein (HDL) cholesterol levels drop significantly.

Estrogenic activities are vital for maintaining the integrity of the vascular endothelium, where atherosclerotic changes begin. Finally, lack of estrogen replacement in the postmenopausal state may predispose women to forms of cardiac muscle disease that are only now beginning to be understood.

Osteoporosis. Hormone deficiencies (beginning as

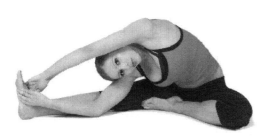

early as age 30) are clearly associated with bone loss and osteoporosis. By the time women reach age 50, they are at a significantly increased risk of an osteoporotic bone fracture. Estrogen deficiency results in increased production of pro-inflammatory cytokines, which cause increased bone breakdown and inflammation. Combined estrogen and androgen (i.e. natural or synthetic) therapy has been shown to increase BMD more than estrogen therapy alone.

Alzheimer's and Dementia. Hormone loss is associated with neuronal degeneration and increased risk of dementia, Alzheimer's disease, and Parkinson's disease. Estrogen stimulates degradation of beta-amyloid protein (noted to accumulate in the brain of Alzheimer's disease patients) by up-regulating production of protective proteins. Deficiencies in pregnenolone and DHEA, which are both neuroprotective hormones, are also linked to reduced memory and brain cell death associated with Alzheimer's disease. These two hormones play an important role in regulating neurotransmitter systems that are involved in learning, stress, depression, addiction, and many other vital functions.

Chapter 10 -
More About the
Importance of Testing

When hormone imbalance is suspected, it is vitally important to properly test your hormone levels. Many doctors and patients dive into "treatment" with synthetic (man-made, unnatural) hormone therapy or bioidentical (natural) hormone therapy. This is like playing "Russian roulette" with your health and body function. Without testing, it is impossible to know what is going on with your

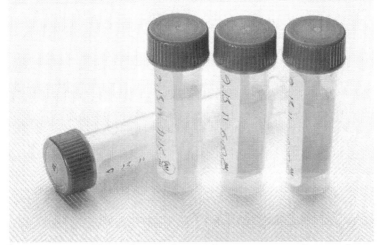

hormones. Treating it in such a manner is madness, but it happens all of the time. Doctors prescribe birth control pills, give hormone creams, and/or give injections or patches every day. All without testing to see what the patient's true hormone levels are at that time.

Proper testing allows for proper treatment and proper results from treatment. It becomes a simple game when you know the players and the rules. Testing allows this to happen. With a reliable and viable test sample, a full picture of the patient's health can be obtained and allow us to fully evaluate the present status and outline an adequate treatment protocol.

Hormone imbalance is a true epidemic in our country. The average American female and male over 35 years of age suffers from some form of hormonal imbalance. With the poor diet, stressful lifestyles and declining popularity of physical exercise, more and more younger men and women are developing hormonal imbalances. The effects of such imbalances increase as we age and become more devastating and harder to treat the longer they go on and the worse they become. Because most of the symptoms come on gradually, it is difficult to figure out initially, until the problems become more pronounced and the hormones become even more imbalanced.

It becomes a vicious cycle that slowly robs you of your energy, your vitality and your life and lifestyle. It also robs your loved ones of their lifestyle. Unless properly diagnosed and evaluated, proper recovery is very difficult to achieve. This is where a properly trained healthcare professional is so important. You will require a doctor who is up-to-date on hormonal function and can discover "subclinical" hormone imbalances, not just "diseased" glands or organs.

Often it is the simplest of signs that indicate hormone imbalance, but these signs are blamed on other factors.

Some of the initial symptoms include:

Fatigue not relieved by rest

Poor sleep

Craving for salt or sugar

Decreased sex drive

Decreased handling of stress

Increased recovery from illness or injury

Light headed, dizzy, or nausea after not eating

Depression

Lack of enjoyment

Weight gain/loss

Anxiety

Digestive disorders

Dry and thin skin

Hair loss

Unexplained headaches

Immune deficiencies

Inability to concentrate

Infections

Liver disorders

Chronic pain

Inflammation

Blood pressure problems

Low body temperature
Hot flashes
Night sweats
Mood swings
Poor memory

PMS
Sleep disorders
Slow metabolism
Yeast overgrowth
Allergies
Chronic fatigue syndrome
Chronic viral infections (EBV, Herpes, etc.)
Migraines
Autoimmune disease
Cancer
Cardiovascular disease
Insomnia
Hypoglycemia
Type II diabetes
Osteoporosis
ADD/ADHD
Irritable bowel disease
Celiac disease
And more...

Quite simply, hormones affect body function. Hormone imbalances affect body functions in a detrimental way.

The more hormones and systems involved and the longer the time that the imbalances have been present, the more symptoms will devastate your life.

Chapter 11 -
Nutrients, Leaky Gut
and Hormones

So, if we really want to get to the root of hormone imbalance and where it starts, you may be quite surprised. With all the environmental issues at work against you can you see now that it is not your fault? Having spent the past 15 years trying to understand how hormones affect every part of the body, mostly in attempt to help myself and the symptoms I suffered, I now have an expert level understanding of what is going on. I have helped thousands of women with hormone imbalance issues.

I want to share with you some of the changes that have happened to us over the past four to six decades that have lead to our hormones having trouble with balance.

Hormones are chemical messengers in our body that direct every process that occurs. You name it. A hormone is responsible for directing the traffic. Sleep. Cholesterol production. Metabolism. Hunger. Feeling full. Feeling happy. Sex drive.... And the list goes on and on.

So getting your hormones balanced is the first step!

When your hormones are balanced you are more likely to have a healthy body weight for getting pregnant and the bottom line is that the female/male reproductive hormones must be in alignment for you to get pregnant!

I believe the first place we have to look for hormone imbalance is a most unlikely place that you may have never thought of...

THE GUT!!!

And by gut I mean the intestines. And this is not only what we eat but how well we absorb the nutrients from what we eat.

How did our intestines or gut get so out of balance?

Well there are lots of reasons. Let's break them down one by one.

- People are eating more junk food than ever before.
- Sugar consumption has sky rocketed.
- Low Fat Diet Fads
- We eat more on the holidays
- Junk food is cheaper
- We sit behind a desk all day
- We eat more with friends and on the weekends
- We don't sleep enough hours to reset our metabolism
- We are consuming more calories than we did even 10 years ago
- Toxins in our environment

I have told patients for years that I suspected pesticides are dangerous but didn't really realize the full extent. I know that certain pesticides resemble estrogen in the body (we call these Xeno-estrogens) and can wreak

hormone

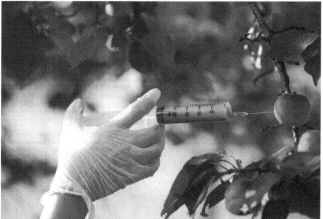

76

irregularities. I also knew that certain chemicals that may be found in "Round-Up" particularly disrupts plant digestive tracts and ours too leading to leaky gut that I will discuss at length as you read on. But here is something interesting.

I have seen a rise in gluten intolerance on food sensitivity testing and knew that it was very problematic for healthy digestion but recently learned that there is something going on with the wheat supply that is not well known by the public.

The issues with our wheat supply go beyond gluten or hybridization, genetically modified or the organic versus non-organic hype, but the problem actually lies in the pesticides on the wheat. Gluten and wheat hybrids have been consumed for many many years and not caused problems. So why all the problems with gluten and wheat now? It's the pesticides!

Standard wheat harvest protocol in the U.S. is to saturate the wheat fields with Round up several days before the combine harvesters harvest the fields to allow for easier and larger harvest as dead withered wheat is easier to plow. Roundup is routinely used by all wheat growers in the U.S. and contains the deadly active ingredient glyphosate, which affects our gastrointestinal absorptive abilities and blocks essential pathways in our livers to clear other toxins we are exposed to. It also disrupts all the pathways found in beneficial gut microbes which are critical for us to able to process, synthesize and absorb critical amino acids and nutrients. Friendly gut bacteria, also called probiotics play a crucial role in all of our digestive processes. Lack of these lead to being essentially malnourished. Glyphosate exposure is slow and insidious over months and years as inflammation gradually gains a foothold in the cellular systems of the body.

The consequences of this systemic inflammation are most may include:

GI Issues
Obesity
Diabetes
Depression
Autism
Infertility
Cancer
Dementia
Heart Disease
Stroke
Heart Attack
And the list goes on and on and on..

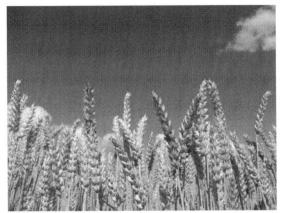 Even if you think you have no trouble digesting wheat, it is still very wise to avoid conventional wheat as much as possible in your diet!

The bottom line is that avoidance of conventional wheat in the United States is absolutely imperative even if you don't currently have a gluten allergy or wheat sensitivity. The increase in the amount of glyphosate applied to wheat closely correlates with the rise of celiac disease and gluten intolerance. These diseases are not just genetic in nature, but also have an environmental cause as not all patient symptoms are alleviated by eliminating gluten from the diet. The effects of deadly glyphosate on your biology are so insidious that lack of symptoms today means literally nothing. If you don't have problems with wheat now, you will in the future if you keep eating conventionally produced, toxic wheat!

Obviously, if you've already developed a sensitivity or allergy to wheat, you must avoid it. Period. *Ok so what do we do about all this? And we may have known all this but what do we do now? And "how does it apply to me?" you may be asking.*

First what I am asking you to do is to simply be aware of what has happened in our country over the past four-six decades that are influencing our environment. This awareness will help you see that you have been duped. Take a deep breath and relax!

After you realize that you are not to blame on what has influenced you then you can begin to take simple action. We will nail this down to a few simple things that you can do to start changing your life and reclaiming your balance.

It is important to keep in mind that it is not some collective moral failure that drives our obesity. All behavior is driven by the underlying biology… and the way the diet and environment have changed has altered the way our brains and hormones work. In other words, these changes have caused malfunctions in the biological systems that are supposed to prevent us from getting fat or getting pregnant. This is the underlying reason for the increased calorie intake and weight gain, NOT a lack of willpower, as some would have you believe.

So where do we go from here?

1. Get some lab work done to see how out of balance you are, this should include
   -Vitamin D, Vitamin B12, iron, kidney and liver testing
   -Full hormone panel (estradiol, estrone, estriol, testosterone, DHEA, cortisol, and a full thyroid panel) for starters
   -Food sensitivity testing
2. Eat out less and limit "junk food"
3. Decrease sugar consumption (read labels as sugar is hidden in everything) if it appears first on a label then it is the MAIN ingredient, BEWARE!
4. Don't concentrate on "Low FAT"- low fat means more preservative and more SUGAR
5. Be aware of Holidays and have a strategy for not binging
6. Be aware that junk food is cheap and make better choices
7. Never drink your calories (water only!)
8. If you work a desk job, especially long hours, take a walk on your lunch break, and get into a regular exercise routine after work

9. Be mindful that when you eat with others you are likely to eat more and watch out for weekend splurges on calories and treats
10. Make an effort to get 6-8 hours of sleep a night.
11. Consume less calories, be aware of portion distortion
12. Don't eat wheat from the U.S. and eat organic pesticide free as much as possible and avoid gluten if at all possible as most people have developed intolerance at this point.

Just being aware that so much has insidiously affected you should make you realize that you are not to blame. Subconscious habits are at play and our environment is making you sick and possibly fat or malnourished and infertile.

A few simple choices can be a game changer.

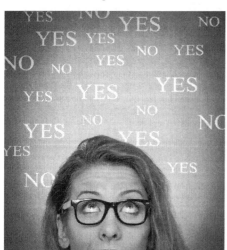

And one more thing that I want to mention is some of the fortification processes that have been implemented and un-implemented. For example iodine, which is primarily necessary for healthy thyroid function was found to be deficient several decades ago and so fortification of this went into the salt supply. You can only imagine what issues this can bring up. And then there is the issue of folate, a vital B-vitamin in every cellular process in the body.

I will go into this in more detail on folate metabolism and preventing birth defects. It was found that as we started eating more junk food and less vegetables that the incidence of spina bifida (a neural tube defect) in newborns went up.

Fortification was noted to be necessary to prevent this but folate was expensive to extract so fortification was made with folic acid, which is cheaper to produce. However, if you have a genetic defect called MTHFR (methylene tetrahydrofolate reductase) the enzyme needed to break down folic acid can't do this properly and you can accumulate homocysteine.

Why understand nutrition?

Nutrition is just one pillar of a full comprehensive design for overall health and metabolic well-being - but it is an essential pillar. Without any one pillar the roof will fall, right? We must begin to think in terms of food not as a social engagement but something that sustains life. EAT

TO LIVE! "Food is eaten to sustain life, provide energy, and promote growth and repair of tissues." - *Macmillan Dictionary*

So, what if you are eating "HEALTHY"? Well most people are eating "healthy" things which are literally making them fat or indirectly or directly infertile. We had a movement in our country a few years ago to go "FAT FREE". We thought simply that "FAT" in foods must make us "FAT". Worse yet we thought that the fat in foods was causing cholesterol or fat in the blood and therefore heart and blood vessel issues leading to stroke and cardiovascular disease. We found that this wasn't true at all. When people stopped eating a lot of fat, do you know what they ate more of... *SUGAR!*

We found that there was more obesity and more heart disease than ever. The sugar caused inflammation through insulin resistance and cortisol increases and adrenal exhaustion. We saw an increase in belly fat and diabetes. We were clearly very wrong. So if that wasn't the answer then what is? I have patients who try to decrease sugar or carbs and still gain weight or can't lose weight. Well I stumbled on to a very straightforward and interesting way to eat which is the basis for sustainable weight loss and wellness forever. Want to hear about it? Of course you do or you wouldn't be reading this.

Well there are foods that you may consider healthy but may not be right for you. *"But how do I know,"* **you might ask.** You probably don't know. But I will tell you not knowing is hurting you. Let me go into an analogy that one of our coaches shared with me.

Imagine you have a car and you have no idea what kind of gas it takes. You go to the pump and you look at the unleaded pump and the diesel fuel pump. Which one do you use? What if you guess and you are wrong? How far will your car go? If you put the wrong fuel in what will be the fix? You have to have the pipes drained right? Well your body is no different. You might think certain foods are healthy but they might not be the right fuel for you. And what do you do if you have the wrong fuel in your tank??? This is the basis for understanding food sensitivities and detox. But first, let me ask you...

Are you experiencing any of these...

1. Digestive issues such as gas, bloating, diarrhea or irritable bowel syndrome (IBS)?
2. Seasonal allergies or asthma?
3. Hormonal imbalances such as menopause symptoms, heavy periods, endometriosis, PMS or PCOS? Low libido? Hot flashes?
4. Diagnosis of an autoimmune disease such as rheumatoid arthritis, Hashimoto's thyroiditis, lupus, psoriasis, or celiac disease?
5. Fatigue? Chronic fatigue?
6. Fibromyalgia? Hurt all the time for no apparent reason?
7. Mood and mind issues such as depression, anxiety, attention deficit issues?
8. Skin issues such as acne, rosacea, or eczema? Itching
9. Diagnosis of yeast infections, or food allergies or intolerances?
10. Memory loss?
11. Cancer, aging, or heart disease?

If you said yes to any of these you probably have food sensitivities. Before we talk about food sensitivities we need to discuss a controversial topic that is very pertinent to our discussion called "Leaky Gut"!

What is LEAKY GUT?

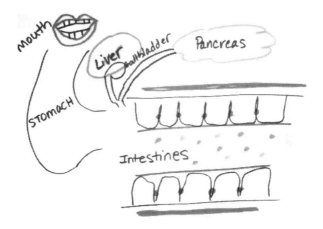

Normal Intestines

Even if you ate veggies from the Garden of Eden, organic and rich with nutrients you would still have to have a perfectly healthy digestive tract, stomach and intestine, to absorb the nutrients from it that you need.

The intestine or gut is naturally permeable to very small molecules in order to absorb these vital nutrients. In fact, regulating intestinal permeability is one of the basic functions of the cells that line the intestinal wall. In sensitive people, gluten can cause the gut cells to release "Zonulin", a protein that can break apart tight junctions in the intestinal lining. Other factors — such as infections, toxins, stress and age — can also cause these tight junctions to break apart.

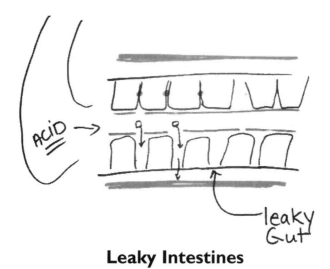

Leaky Intestines

Once these tight junctions get broken apart, you have a leaky gut. When your gut is leaky, things like toxins, microbes, undigested food particles, and more can escape from your intestines and travel throughout your body via your bloodstream. Your immune system marks these "foreign invaders" as pathogens and attacks them.

So, what causes leaky gut?

The main culprits are toxins (pesticides) unhealthy junk foods with preservatives and sugar, infections, gluten, a protein found in wheat, and inflammatory foods like dairy, sugar (which feeds the yeast in the gut) and excessive alcohol is suspected as well. The most common infectious causes are yeast, intestinal parasites, and small intestine bacterial overgrowth. Toxins come in the form of medications, like Motrin, Advil, steroids, antibiotics, and acid-reducing drugs, and environmental toxins like Mercury, pesticides and BPA from plastics. Stress, leaking stomach acid into the intestines, hormone changes and aging also contributes to a leaky gut.

The good news is there's a solution to healing leaky gut.

To keep it simple, here are some basics to start with...

- Remove foods and factors that damage the gut such as sugar, grains, dairy and GMO foods, non-organic foods, acidic substances like coffee and drugs like ibuprofen, acid reducers, and non-essential antibiotics and ask your doctor about medications that you may not need. **Get food allergies tested!** Identify your specific food sensitivities and remove them from your diet. A 21-day detox protocol of eliminating the foods you are sensitive is essential to healing the gut. If your car had diesel fuel in it and it was an unleaded gas engine you would need to remove the wrong fuel from the line.

- Replace with healing foods like Bone Broth, Fermented Vegetables and Coconut and Super seeds like Chia seeds, flaxseeds, and hemp seeds (as long as they are not on your food sensitivity/allergy list). Also, consuming foods that have anti-inflammatory Omega-3 fats are beneficial such as grass-fed beef, lamb, and wild-caught fish like salmon.

- Repair with specific supplements, these include specific amino acids, magnesium, digestive enzymes, probiotics and anti inflammatories. Certain amino acids act like "gut spackling" and protects and coats the intestinal wall, and acts as an anti-inflammatory as well as does Aloe-Vera licorice, Reservatrol and Turmeric among many we recommend. Digestive enzymes ensure that food is fully digested, decreasing the chance of undigested foods traversing the leaky gut and causing immune response. Magnesium relaxes smooth muscle in the gut keeping things moving.

- Rebalance with probiotics, last but most importantly this is THE Vital Part to Healing Your Gut. You must rebalance with the right probiotics. Many on the market have the wrong ratio or have ingredients that may make your issues worse. It is essential to get at least 100 billion units the right ratio of bacteria.

Food allergy/sensitivity testing is a vital piece to the balance that the system is seeking as well as supplements that heal the digestive process.

When I first learned about food sensitivities, I was working with a chiropractor. He was using food sensitivities for joint pain, chronic pain, fibromyalgia and all the maladies that most patients seek out a chiropractor for. I have always been amazed at how chiropractors know things that traditional doctors don't. They don't have a prescription pad at their fingertips so they have to learn what "works" if they really want to get results.

He taught me the basics of how certain foods trigger inflammation in the body and this inflammation spreads to joints, muscles, and tendons causing pain but more than that this inflammation is in the blood vessels and causing more insidious disease that may end up in heart disease, strokes, cancer autoimmune disease and possible cancer. These end points resulting in possible death. I watched as he order test after test and got amazing results.

I had a patient who came in one day with obvious hormone imbalance and terrible fibromyalgia. I was thinking it was the hormone imbalance but after I clearly corrected that she still continued to have pain. So I did what my chiropractor friend recommended and ordered the food sensitivity test. She returned for the results and I explained how it worked. She seemed skeptical and we scheduled her a three-month follow up appointment. Fast forward to that appointment.

I watched her walk into the room. Without limping. Without her cane and without obvious distress. She had a glow about her that I could not explain. Her skin was brighter and her mood lighter. She took a seat and although her physical state was remarkably improved she had an energy about her that was confusing. She smiled softly. I noticed that she appeared about twenty pounds lighter than I had seen her last.

"Looks like you are doing much better!" I exclaimed. *"Oh, I am, but..."* she said.

"But what?!?" I looked puzzled. She smiled, *"I am doing amazing. I have lost twenty pounds. My joints do not hurt and the muscle pain is ninety percent improved. I have followed the food sensitivity test and had remarkable results. I am quite upset, however."*

"Go on...", I encouraged her.

"I am very frustrated because over six years ago, a doctor did the food sensitivity test on me and recommended that I make dietary changes. I thought he was crazy. I'm upset because I have suffered for over six years with these symptoms and the answer was so simple. Right in front of me! It took you with your confidence to convince me, or maybe just the tremendous suffering to finally take the leap and make some changes. I am so grateful for the change in my life but frustrated that I didn't listen sooner and I have suffered so much all these years."

I was amazed as she told me this and I took it to heart. I started using the test on everyone that I could think of with chronic pain. I never really thought about the weight loss as I thought that was just an effect of her eating less.

93

Fast forward a few years and many patient success stories (all the while not acknowledging the effects of the weight loss) and I had a husband and wife come in the office one day. He was having terrible gastrointestinal symptoms. His wife was very frustrated and felt that it was affecting his health. He had terrible gas, bloating, and constipation alternating with diarrhea every time he ate.

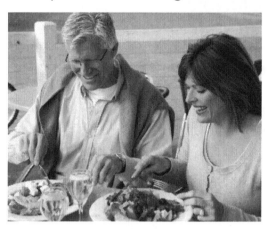

He had been diagnosed with "IBS" or irritable bowel syndrome and put on many prescription medications that simply did not help. It was affecting his work, his home life and his sleep. He was in terrible pain all over and his hormones were all out of balance by blood test. I recommended the food sensitivity test.

He was more than willing to comply as no one had helped him thus far. We discussed dietary substitutions and he returned for his follow up three months later. He was thrilled. He had lost thirty pounds and he was so happy to be empowered to know what foods caused his pain and distress.

He had avoided them strictly and adhered to the recommendations. All was well... Or so I thought. His wife was quite upset. She sat in the opposite chair with a very closed off energy, her arms crossed about her chest and a stern look on her face. I turned to her and said, *"Aren't you happy that he is doing so well?"*

"Oh yes!" She replied. *"He is doing great, but since I have been cooking for him I have gained twenty pounds!"*

I was confused. *"How could cooking for him, the clean and healthy foods that I recommended while avoiding his trigger foods have caused her to gain weight? Was something else going on?"* And then I realized that maybe there was a recurring theme to this weight loss I had witnessed in patients who had complied with the dietary recommendations. Maybe hers were different? And so I recommended that we test her, to which she was reluctant but agreed.

To my amazement, her list of foods that she was sensitive too was almost completely opposite of his. I realized in that moment the power of this food sensitivity program.

She was willing to try to make meals separately for each of them and at her three month follow she had lost the extra twenty she had gained plus ten more pounds. *"Holy Crap!" I thought! "This is huge!"*

I had personally gained almost eighty pounds on synthetic hormones after my hysterectomy and when I went on bioidentical hormones and started exercising I had lost all but the last fifteen or twenty pounds. I thought to myself that I would do the test and see if this really worked. So I did... **and it did**!

I am down to 130 pounds and follow my list very closely and feel wonderful. Years of stomach pain and IBS and struggling with my weight were gone. I have since used this strategy on thousands of patients and get consistent results as long as the patient understand, believes and adheres to the test and follows it. I have been giddy with the discovery until I went to my annual continuing education courses at the anti-aging conference and learned that many doctors all over the world are using the food sensitivity results for weight loss. *I had patted myself on the back for discovering this and felt quite deflated in that I did not really discover anything at all.*

We have created a whole program around food sensitivities and continue to get incredible results.

"So how does this work?" **You may ask.**

The inability to tolerate certain foods also known as sensitivity or intolerance, induces chronic activation of the immune system. Free radicals are produced and mediators of inflammation. This inflammation has been linked to countless chronic conditions, including: digestive disorders, migraines, obesity, chronic fatigue, attention deficit issues, aching joints, skin disorders, arthritis and many more.

This inflammation induces a cortisol response from the adrenal glands which ultimately leads to unwanted belly fat. (See section on hormones.)

How does food sensitivity differ from classic food allergies?

True or immediate food allergies refer to foods that trigger the immune system to acutely produce massive amounts of the chemical histamine that leads to anaphylaxis or a potentially fatal condition that may cause the throat and esophagus (swallowing tube) to swell, cutting off air from the lungs, or may simply cause hives, skin rashes, and other non-life-threatening reactions.

97

This type of reaction is called a hypersensitivity reaction, caused by the degranulation of mast cells or basophiles that is mediated by Immunoglobulin E (IgE). This happens within minutes. Then there is a delayed reaction that can take up to 3 days to appear. This is mediated by the part of the immune system called IgG. Food allergies are divided into two major categories: immediate and delayed. Delayed can take up to 72 hours to appear.

Some people get confused about food allergies versus sensitivities. When we talk of the delayed response we often refer to this as a "sensitivity" or "food intolerance".

Non-IgE-mediated food hypersensitivity (food intolerance) is more chronic, less acute, less obvious in its presentation, and often more difficult to diagnose than a food allergy. Symptoms of food intolerance vary greatly, and can be mistaken for the symptoms of a food allergy.

Food intolerance can present with symptoms affecting the skin, respiratory tract, gastrointestinal tract either individually or in combination. On the skin may include skin rashes, itching, hives, swelling and chronic eczema. Respiratory tract symptoms can include a stuffy nose, sinus infections, asthma, and cough among many.

Gastrointestinal symptoms may include ulcers in the mouth, reflux or chest pain (heart burn), abdominal cramps, nausea, gas, bloating, intermittent diarrhea or constipation (irritable bowel symptoms-IBS) and vomiting or even prolonged gastritis, bleeding, hemorrhoids, ulcers and chronic gastrointestinal pain.

Other symptoms include headaches, joint and muscle pains and lead to more insidious disease from the inflammation like cancer, aging and cardiovascular disease (heart attacks and strokes).

If you have any symptoms you can test to see if you have food sensitivities.

Fifteen/Fifteen Rule Test

One quick and dirty test you can do is to get a stop watch and monitor your pulse for one minute. If you eat something you are sensitive to your pulse will go up fifteen or more beats within fifteen minutes. The problem with this is that it is sensitive but not specific. You won't know what food triggered you. If you eat multiple foods it could be any one of them. You can experiment with different isolated foods to do this test. The problem is that it has to be a pretty severe sensitivity to trigger a response this quickly. Some of the milder triggers may take up to three days to trigger this response.

Elimination Diet

One other way you can try is elimination diet but this can be tricky because often when someone gives up one food they often eat more of something else they could be triggered by.

Blood Test

The other option and a much more reasonable option is just to have your blood tested. This is sensitive, specific and spot on every time. How do you test for them?

This is measured as IgG, unlike IgE (immediate response/allergy). This is a delayed response by the immune system. To verify if you have an IgG food intolerance a simple blood test can be done to identify 100 to 200 foods. A blood sample is taken, the lab technician identifies delayed onset allergies by observing how white blood cells and red blood cells react if they are exposed to selected foods.

Red and white blood cell samples literally explode when allergens are introduced. What is also excellent around the allergy test is that the test will not be tied to detecting food intolerances; it may also identify reactions to artificial additives, antibiotics, environmental chemicals, and pharmacological ingredients.

The process measures the amount of response as well as if there is a response of your white blood cell antibodies (IgG) to protein substance (antigens) in the specific foods tested.

This is a sample food allergy test panel from Alletess, the company we use most often.

TEST	SCORE	CLASS		TEST	SCORE	CLASS	
ALMOND	0.179	0		LETTUCE	0.158	0	
APPLE	0.159	0		LOBSTER	0.170	0	
ASPARAGUS	0.175	0		MALT	0.157	0	
AVOCADO	0.157	0		MILK (COW'S)	0.310	2	**
BANANA	0.161	0		MUSHROOM	0.211	1	*
BARLEY	0.263	1	*	MUSTARD	0.168	0	
BASIL	0.170	0		NUTRA SWEET	0.157	0	
BAY LEAF	0.160	0		OAT	0.166	0	
BEAN (GREEN)	0.172	0		OLIVE (GREEN)	0.155	0	
BEAN (LIMA)	0.176	0		ONION	0.161	0	
BEAN (PINTO)	0.289	1	*	ORANGE	0.172	0	
BEEF	0.168	0		OREGANO	0.155	0	
BLUEBERRY	0.150	0		PEA	0.182	0	
BRAN	0.155	0		PEACH	0.148	0	
BROCCOLI	0.222	1	*	PEANUT	0.151	0	
CABBAGE	0.163	0		PEAR	0.139	0	
CANTALOUPE	0.190	0		PEPPER (BLACK)	0.151	0	
CARROT	0.172	0		PEPPER (CHILI)	0.153	0	
CASHEW	0.213	1	*	PEPPER (GREEN)	0.151	0	
CAULIFLOWER	0.206	1	*	PINEAPPLE	0.266	1	*
CELERY	0.149	0		PORK	0.127	0	
CHEESE (CHEDDAR)	0.144	0		POTATO (SWEET)	0.145	0	
CHEESE (COTTAGE)	0.141	0		POTATO (WHITE)	0.147	0	
CHEESE (SWISS)	0.146	0		RICE	0.137	0	
CHICKEN	0.155	0		RYE	0.206	1	*
CINNAMON	0.122	0		SAFFLOWER	0.149	0	
CLAM	0.139	0		SALMON	0.184	0	
COCOA	0.209	1	*	SCALLOP	0.146	0	
COCONUT	0.173	0		SESAME	0.139	0	
CODFISH	0.151	0		SHRIMP	0.159	0	
COFFEE	0.266	1	*	SOLE	0.190	0	
COLA	0.144	0		SOYBEAN	0.144	0	
CORN	0.141	0		SPINACH	0.143	0	
CRAB	0.231	1	*	SQUASH	0.145	0	
CUCUMBER	0.159	0		STRAWBERRY	0.142	0	
DILL	0.151	0		SUGAR (CANE)	0.134	0	
EGG WHITE	0.290	1	*	SUNFLOWER (SEED)	0.136	0	
EGG YOLK	0.193	0		SWORDFISH	0.147	0	
EGGPLANT	0.161	0		TEA (BLACK)	0.163	0	
GARLIC	0.141	0		TOMATO	0.156	0	
GINGER	0.256	1	*	TUNA	0.200	1	*
GLUTEN	0.319	2	**	TURKEY	0.151	0	
GRAPE	0.150	0		WALNUT (BLACK)	0.166	0	
GRAPEFRUIT	0.161	0		WATERMELON	0.162	0	
HADDOCK	0.147	0		WHEAT	0.310	2	**

You can see on this test that the foods in red have triggered an IgG reaction in this patient and it is rated 1, 2 or 3. The higher the number the more reactive the patient is to that food. 3 is the worst, or 3 stars or the higher the number the worse the reaction.

I recommend doing a 21-day detox in which you avoid all foods in red and afterward in the rotation schedule you rotate foods with a 1 or 2, every 3-5 days and avoid 3s. The rationale for this is that it takes approximately 3 days to develop a new IgG antibody/antigen protein reaction, giving your body time to reset the inflammatory response.

Other Important Supplements:

Vitamin D. Vitamin D confers significant protective effects against breast cancer. In a study, women with higher vitamin D levels had a nearly 70% reduction in their risk of breast cancer compared to women with the lowest levels. Vitamin D helps prevent mutated cells from becoming malignant and even induces cancer cell death (apoptosis). Human studies show that doses of 1100 IU vitamin D daily plus calcium result in a 60% risk reduction for developing any cancer, compared with placebo.

Nutrients to Support Hormonal Balance and Healthy Hormonal Metabolism

Vitamin D3: 5000 – 8000 IU daily

Omega-3 fatty acids (from fish): 2000 – 6000 mg daily

Calcium D-glucarate: 200 – 600 mg daily

DHEA: 25 – 50 mg daily (depending on blood test results)

Pregnenolone: 50 – 100 mg daily (depending on blood test results)

Progesterone cream: Per label directions

Reserveratrol, Tumeric and Gluthathione can help block the production of damaging quinones

DIM – diindolylmethane-A phytonutrient and plant indole found in cruciferous vegetables including broccoli, Brussel sprouts, cabbage, cauliflower and kale, with potential antiandrogenic and antineoplastic activities. As a dimmer of indole-3-carbinol, diindolylmethane (DIM) promotes beneficial estrogen metabolism in both sexes by reducing the levels of 16-hydroxy estrogen metabolites and increasing the formation of 2-hydroxy estrogen metabolites, resulting in increased antioxidant activity.

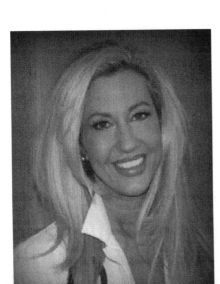

Summary: When it Comes to Hormones

1. Don't assume
2. Understand your body, listen to it
3. You are right to be reluctant about artificial HRT
4. When supplementing with bioidentical hormones make sure you get tested so you know what you actually need and then work with someone knowledgeable that can prescribe only what you need but in adequate amounts without using excess amounts
5. Focus on getting in balance with all your hormones not just the ovarian (sex steroid hormones) and this includes thyroid, adrenal, insulin, etc.
6. Go to the source of imbalance, get food sensitivity testing and do an efficient detox
7. Start your amazing, wonderful, fabulous life of having your hormones balanced, feeling good, sexy and back in CONTROL!

34402266R00060

Made in the USA
San Bernardino, CA
27 May 2016